FIGHT AGAINST FATTY LIVER CIRRHOSIS

All that You Need to Know About Fatty Liver

Dr. Christine Howells

Contents

CHAPTER ONE 4
- All that You Need to Know About Fatty Liver 4
- Manifestations of greasy liver 6

CHAPTER TWO 10
- Reasons for greasy liver 10
- Less regular causes include: 12
- Diagnosing of greasy liver 13

CHAPTER THREE 14
- Restorative history 14
- Physical test 15
- Blood tests 16
- Imaging examines 18

CHAPTER FOUR 20
- Liver biopsy 20
- Treatment for greasy liver 21
- Home cures 23

CHAPTER FIVE 26
- Diet for greasy liver illness 26
- Kinds of greasy liver illness 28
- Nonalcoholic greasy liver ailment (NAFLD) .. 29

Nonalcoholic steatohepatitis (NASH)...........30
Intense greasy liver of pregnancy (AFLP).....31
Alcoholic greasy liver ailment (ALFD)...........33
Alcoholic steatohepatitis (ASH)....................34
CHAPTER SIX 36
Hazard factors..36
Phases of greasy liver..................................38
Picture..40
Aversion 41
Viewpoint...42
THE END 45

CHAPTER ONE

All that You Need to Know About Fatty Liver

Greasy liver is otherwise called hepatic steatosis. It happens when fat develops in the liver. Having modest quantities of fat in your liver is ordinary, however an excessive amount of can turn into a medical issue.

Your liver is the second biggest organ in your body. It helps process supplements from nourishment and beverages and channels unsafe substances from your blood.

A lot of fat in your liver can cause liver aggravation, which can harm your liver and make scarring. In extreme cases, this scarring can prompt liver disappointment.

At the point when greasy liver creates in somebody who drinks a ton of liquor, it's known as alcoholic greasy liver illness (AFLD).

In somebody who doesn't drink a great deal of liquor, it's known as non-alcoholic greasy liver sickness (NAFLD). As per specialists in the World Journal of Gastroenterology, NAFLD influences up to 25 to 30 percent of individuals in the United States and Europe.

Manifestations of greasy liver

By and large, greasy liver causes no observable indications. However, you may feel tired or experience distress or torment in the upper right half of your belly.

A few people with greasy liver infection create intricacies, including liver scarring. Liver scarring is known as liver fibrosis. On the off chance that you create serious liver fibrosis, it's known as cirrhosis.

Cirrhosis may cause manifestations, for example,

- *loss of hunger*

- *weight misfortune*

- *weakness*

- *fatigue*

- *nosebleeds*

- *itchy skin*

- *yellow skin and eyes*

- *web-like groups of veins under your skin*

- *abdominal torment*

- *abdominal growing*

- *swelling of your legs*

- *breast development in men*

- *confusion*

Cirrhosis is a conceivably perilous condition. Get the data you have to perceive and oversee it.

CHAPTER TWO

Reasons for greasy liver

Greasy liver creates when your body delivers an excess of fat or doesn't utilize fat productively enough. The overabundance fat is put away in liver cells, where it gathers and causes greasy liver illness.

This development of fat can be brought about by an assortment of things.

For instance, drinking an excessive amount of liquor can cause alcoholic greasy liver infection. This is the primary phase of liquor related liver ailment.

In individuals who don't drink a great deal of liquor, the reason for greasy liver sickness is less clear.

At least one of the accompanying variables may assume a job:

- *obesity*

- *high glucose*

- *insulin opposition*

• *high levels of fat, particularly triglycerides, in your blood*

Less regular causes include:

• *pregnancy*

• *rapid weight reduction*

• *some sorts of diseases, for example, hepatitis C*

• *side impacts from certain sorts of meds, for example, methotrexate (Trexall), tamoxifen (Nolvadex), amiodorone*

(Pacerone), and valproic corrosive (Depakote)

- *exposure to specific poisons*

Certain qualities may likewise raise your danger of creating greasy liver.

Diagnosing of greasy liver

To analyze greasy liver, your PCP will take your therapeutic history, lead a physical test, and request at least one tests.

CHAPTER THREE

Restorative history

In the event that your primary care physician speculates that you may have greasy liver, they will probably ask you inquiries about:

• your family therapeutic history, including any history of liver illness

• your liquor utilization and other way of life propensities

• any ailments that you may have

- *any meds that you may take*

- *recent changes in your wellbeing*

On the off chance that you've been encountering exhaustion, loss of craving, or other unexplained side effects, let your primary care physician know.

Physical test

To check for liver aggravation, your primary care physician may palpate or push on your stomach area. In the event that your liver is broadened, they may have the option to feel it.

Be that as it may, it's feasible for your liver to be aroused without being expanded. Your primary care physician probably won't have the option to tell if your liver is aroused by contact.

Blood tests

Much of the time, greasy liver illness is analyzed after blood tests show raised liver compounds. For instance, your primary care physician may arrange the alanine aminotransferase test (ALT) and aspartate aminotransferase test (AST) to check your liver chemicals.

These tests may be suggested in the event that you've created signs or side effects of liver ailment, or they may be requested as a feature of routine blood work.

Raised liver compounds are an indication of liver irritation. Greasy liver infection is one potential reason for liver irritation, however it's not alone.

In the event that you test positive for raised liver compounds, your primary care physician will probably arrange extra tests to recognize the reason for the irritation.

Imaging examines

Your primary care physician may utilize at least one of the accompanying imaging tests to check for abundance fat or different issues with your liver:

- *ultrasound test*

- *CT examine*

- *MRI filter*

They may likewise arrange a test known as vibration-controlled transient elastography (VCTE, FibroScan). This test utilizes low-

recurrence sound waves to quantify liver firmness. It can help check for scarring.

CHAPTER FOUR

Liver biopsy

A liver biopsy is viewed as the most ideal approach to decide the seriousness of liver infection.

During a liver biopsy, a specialist will embed a needle into your liver and expel a bit of tissue for assessment. They will give you a nearby analgesic to decrease the torment.

This test can help decide whether you have greasy liver illness, just as liver scarring.

Treatment for greasy liver

At present, no meds have been endorsed to treat greasy liver infection. More research is expected to create and test prescriptions to treat this condition.

By and large, way of life changes can help switch greasy liver illness. For instance, your PCP may encourage you to:

- *limit or maintain a strategic distance from liquor*

- *take steps to get in shape*

- *make changes to your eating regimen*

In the event that you've created difficulties, your primary care physician may suggest extra medications. To treat cirrhosis, for instance, they may endorse:

- *lifestyle changes*

- *medications*

- *surgery*

Cirrhosis can prompt liver disappointment. In the event that you create liver disappointment, you may require a liver transplant.

Home cures

Way of life changes are the primary line treatment for greasy liver illness. Contingent upon your present condition and way of life propensities, it may help to:

- *lose weight*

- *reduce your liquor admission*

- *eat a supplement rich eating routine that is low in*

overabundance calories, immersed fat, and trans fats

- *get in any event 30 minutes of activity most days of the week*

As per the Mayo Clinic, some proof proposes that nutrient E enhancements may help anticipate or treat liver harm brought about by greasy liver infection. In any case, more research is required. There are some wellbeing dangers related with devouring an excess of nutrient E.

Continuously converse with your primary care physician before you attempt another enhancement or normal cure. A few enhancements or regular cures may put weight on your liver or communicate with meds you're taking.

CHAPTER FIVE

Diet for greasy liver illness

On the off chance that you have greasy liver ailment, your primary care physician may urge you to modify your eating regimen to help treat the condition and lower your danger of confusions. For instance, they may encourage you to do the accompanying:

• *Eat an eating routine that is wealthy in plant-based nourishments, including organic products, vegetables, vegetables, and entire grains.*

- *Limit your utilization of refined sugars, for example, desserts, white rice, white bread, other refined grain items.*

- *Limit your utilization of immersed fats, which are found in red meat and numerous other creature items.*

- *Avoid Trans fats, which are available in many handled nibble nourishments.*

- *Avoid liquor.*

Your primary care physician may urge you to slice calories from your eating regimen to get thinner. Get familiar with a portion of the other dietary changes that may assist you with overseeing greasy liver sickness.

Kinds of greasy liver illness

There are two fundamental kinds of greasy liver ailment: nonalcoholic and alcoholic.

Nonalcoholic greasy liver illness (NAFLD) incorporates straightforward nonalcoholic greasy liver, nonalcoholic steatohepatitis (NASH), and intense greasy liver of pregnancy (AFLP).

Alcoholic greasy liver illness (AFLD) incorporates straightforward AFLD and alcoholic steatohepatitis (ASH).

Nonalcoholic greasy liver ailment (NAFLD)

Nonalcoholic greasy liver ailment (NAFLD) happens when fat develops in the liver of individuals who don't drink a great deal of liquor.

On the off chance that you have abundance fat in your liver and no history of overwhelming liquor use, your primary care physician may determine you to have NAFLD.

In the event that there's no irritation or different inconveniences alongside the development of fat, the condition is known as straightforward nonalcoholic greasy liver.

Nonalcoholic steatohepatitis (NASH)

Nonalcoholic steatohepatitis (NASH) is a sort of NAFLD. It happens when a development of overabundance fat in the liver is joined by liver irritation.

In the event that you have overabundance fat in your liver, your liver is excited, and you have no history of overwhelming liquor use, your primary care physician may determine you to have NASH.

At the point when left untreated, NASH can cause scarring of your liver. In serious cases, this can prompt cirrhosis and liver disappointment.

Intense greasy liver of pregnancy (AFLP)

Intense greasy liver of pregnancy (AFLP) is an uncommon yet genuine complexity of pregnancy. The careful reason is obscure.

When AFLP creates, it typically shows up in the third trimester of pregnancy. Whenever left untreated, it presents genuine wellbeing dangers to the mother and developing infant.

In case you're determined to have AFLP, your primary care physician will need to convey your child as quickly as time permits. You may need to get follow-up care for a few days after you conceive an offspring.

Your liver wellbeing will probably come back to typical inside half a month of conceiving an offspring.

Alcoholic greasy liver ailment (ALFD)

Drinking a great deal of liquor harms the liver. At the point when it's harmed, the liver can't separate fat appropriately. This can make fat develop, which is known as alcoholic greasy liver.

Alcoholic greasy liver ailment (ALFD) is the most punctual phase of liquor related liver malady.

On the off chance that there's no irritation or different complexities alongside the development of fat, the condition is known as straightforward alcoholic greasy liver.

Alcoholic steatohepatitis (ASH)

Alcoholic steatohepatitis (ASH) is a sort of AFLD. It happens when a development of abundance fat in the liver is joined by liver aggravation. This is otherwise called alcoholic hepatitis.

On the off chance that you have abundance fat in your liver, your liver is excited, and you drink a great deal of liquor, your primary care physician may determine you to have ASH.

In the event that it's not treated appropriately, ASH can cause scarring of your liver. Serious liver scarring is known as cirrhosis. It can prompt liver disappointment.

To treat alcoholic greasy liver, it's critical to keep away from liquor. On the off chance that you have liquor addiction, or liquor use issue, your primary care physician may prescribe guiding or different medications. Peruse increasingly about the impacts that liquor can have on your body.

CHAPTER SIX

Hazard factors

Drinking high measures of liquor puts you at expanded danger of creating greasy liver.

You may likewise be at elevated hazard on the off chance that you:

- *are large*

- *have insulin opposition*

- *have type 2 diabetes*

- *have polycystic ovary disorder*

- *are pregnant*

- *have a background marked by specific contaminations, for example, hepatitis C*

- *take certain drugs, for example, methotrexate (Trexall), tamoxifen (Nolvadex), amiodorone (Pacerone), and valproic corrosive (Depakote)*

- *have elevated cholesterol levels*

- *have high triglyceride levels*

- *have high glucose levels*

- *have metabolic disorder*

In the event that you have a family ancestry of greasy liver ailment, you're bound to create it yourself.

Phases of greasy liver

Greasy liver can advance through four phases:

* *Simple greasy liver. There is a development of overabundance fat in the liver.*

* *Steatohepatitis. Notwithstanding abundance fat, there is irritation in the liver.*

* *Fibrosis. Aggravation in the liver has caused scarring.*

* *Cirrhosis. Scarring of the liver has gotten far reaching.*

Cirrhosis is a possibly dangerous condition that can cause liver disappointment. It might be irreversible. That is the reason it's so essential to keep it from creating in any case.

To help prevent greasy liver from advancing and causing difficulties, pursue your primary care physician's suggested treatment plan.

Picture

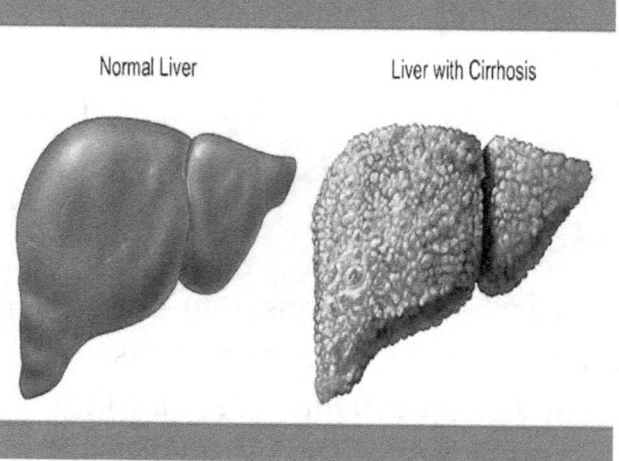

Aversion

To avert greasy liver and its potential intricacies, it's imperative to pursue a sound way of life.

- *Limit or maintain a strategic distance from liquor.*

- *Maintain a solid weight.*

- *Eat a supplement rich eating regimen that is low in soaked fats, trans fats, and refined starches.*

- *Take steps to control your glucose, triglyceride levels, and cholesterol levels.*

• Follow your PCP's prescribed treatment plan for diabetes, in the event that you have it.

• Aim for at any rate 30 minutes of activity most days of the week.

Making these strides can likewise help improve your general wellbeing.

Viewpoint
As a rule, it's conceivable to switch greasy liver through way of life changes. These

progressions may help anticipate liver harm and scarring.

The condition can cause irritation, harm to your liver, and possibly irreversible scarring if it's not treated. Serious liver scarring is known as cirrhosis.

In the event that you create cirrhosis, it expands your danger of liver malignancy and liver disappointment. These confusions can be deadly.

For the best result, it's critical to pursue your primary care physician's suggested treatment plan and practice a general sound way of life.

On the off chance that you have overabundance fat in your liver, your liver is kindled, and you have no history of overwhelming liquor use, your primary care physician may determine you to have NASH. At the point when left untreated, NASH can cause scarring of your liver. In serious cases, this can prompt cirrhosis and liver disappointment.

THE END

www.ingramcontent.com/pod-product-compliance
Lightning Source LLC
Chambersburg PA
CBHW070840220526
45466CB00002B/834